GUIDE TWO:

MASTERING MOISTURE

*From Root to Tip: A Growing Hands
Guide for Natural Hair*

BY CONSTANCE HUNTER

For permissions, inquiries, or additional resources, please contact:

Pre'Vail Natural Hair Salon

www.prevailyournatural.com | prevailyournatural@gmail.com

This book is intended for informational and educational purposes only and should serve as a general guide to understanding and improving natural hair health. While the methods and recommendations provided are based on expertise in natural hair care and trichology, they are not intended to replace professional medical or dermatological advice.

If you are experiencing severe scalp conditions, excessive hair loss, or other persistent issues, it is strongly recommended that you consult a licensed dermatologist or a professional cosmetologist specializing in scalp and hair health. A trained professional can assess underlying causes and provide personalized treatment plans tailored to your specific needs.

By using the information in this book, the reader acknowledges that the author and publisher are not responsible for individual outcomes. Readers should exercise their own discretion when applying the suggested practices.

First Edition: 2025

ISBN:

Paperback: 978-1-968134-02-0

Ebook: 978-1-968134-11-2

Printed in **USA**

ABOUT THE AUTHOR

As a certified trichologist and natural hair care educator, I specialize in helping individuals discover what's truly possible for their hair—especially when they've been told otherwise.

My passion lies in witnessing transformation—that moment when someone realizes their hair can be healthy, strong, and free. With a deep understanding of the science behind hair and scalp health, I strive to provide clarity, comfort, and actionable solutions. My training equips me to assess and guide care for a wide range of concerns, from common challenges like dandruff and dryness to complex conditions such as alopecia areata, scalp psoriasis, and CCCA.

But my work goes beyond diagnosis or technique. I believe in education, empowerment, and helping clients build routines that nourish their crown from root to tip. This includes learning to read labels, choosing products with purpose, avoiding harmful styling practices, and embracing care that fits their lifestyle and values.

While I offer expert insight from the field of trichology, I'm not a medical doctor. Hair and scalp symptoms can sometimes signal deeper health issues. That's why I encourage a holistic approach—and, when necessary, consulting licensed healthcare professionals for comprehensive support.

In this series, you'll find guidance rooted in science, experience, and care. My hope is that it not only helps you understand your hair better but also love it more, trust it more, and grow with it in ways you never thought possible.

Your hair is not the problem—you just needed the right guide.

DEDICATION

For the one tired of dryness, breakage, and confusion:

Your hair isn't thirsty for more product—
It's thirsty for care that truly understands it.

OVERVIEW

Moisture is the heartbeat of healthy natural hair. *Mastering Moisture* teaches you what your hair truly needs to stay hydrated, soft, and strong—without the stress or confusion. You'll learn how to care for your hair based on its unique porosity and needs, rather than relying on trial and error.

Say goodbye to dryness and hello to long-lasting hydration. This guide helps you create a moisture strategy that delivers real results—from wash day to every day.

SERIES INTRODUCTION

Welcome to *From Root to Tip: A Growing Hands Guide for Natural Hair*

This series was created with one goal in mind: to give you what's been missing—not just products, not just trends, but truth, support, and real guidance for real people who are ready to finally understand and care for their natural hair from the inside out.

For years, we've been taught to manage, fix, or fight our hair. But here, we're doing something different. We're returning to care—not control. To confidence. To consistency. To choice.

Each guide in this series is built as a step in your journey. They can be read in order or on their own, depending on where you are in your process. Whether you're just starting out, rebuilding your relationship with your hair, or deepening your understanding, this space is for you.

I've written these guides from my hands—growing hands that have touched, healed, protected, and restored countless crowns. Now, I offer that care to you.

This isn't just about hair. It's about healing. It's about reclaiming your rhythm, your confidence, and your beauty—from root to tip.

Let's begin.

WHAT YOU WILL LEARN

- The difference between moisture and hydration (and why it matters)

- How porosity affects your hair's ability to retain moisture

- Layering techniques: LOC vs. LCO—and how to choose the right method

- Signs of moisture overload vs. protein deficiency

- How to prevent dryness between wash days

- The role of water, leave-ins, oils, and creams in your moisture plan

WHAT YOU'LL WALK AWAY WITH

- A consistent moisture routine tailored to your hair's porosity

- Softer, stronger, and more manageable hair

- Fewer dry-day frustrations and longer-lasting results

- Confidence in caring for your curls with clarity—not confusion

TABLE OF CONTENTS

INTRODUCTION

Dry hair isn't a personal failure—it's a signal.

In *Mastering Moisture*, we uncover the truth about what it really takes to keep natural hair hydrated. You'll explore porosity, layering methods like LOC and LCO, and how to tell the difference between dryness and dehydration. Plus, you'll learn how to balance moisture with protein for the perfect combination of softness and strength.

This guide is all about making moisture *make sense*—so you can stop guessing and start giving your hair exactly what it needs to thrive.

LESSON 1:
SCALP HEALTH AND HYGIENE

Maintaining a healthy scalp is the cornerstone of achieving and sustaining beautiful, vibrant natural hair. As a stylist, understanding the importance of scalp health and mastering effective cleansing techniques are essential skills for delivering exceptional care to clients.

This lesson explores why scalp health matters, highlights effective cleansing practices, and provides product recommendations that support a healthy scalp and natural hair.

The Importance of a Healthy Scalp

The scalp serves as the foundation for hair growth, making its health critical to the overall condition of your hair. A well-maintained scalp fosters optimal hair growth, alleviates common issues like dandruff and itching, and enhances the hair's appearance and vitality.

1. **Hair Growth:** A healthy scalp creates the ideal environment for hair follicles to flourish. Proper blood circulation, balanced sebum production, and minimal buildup of dead skin cells all contribute to stronger, more resilient hair growth. When the scalp is well-cared for, hair follicles can function at their best, resulting in thicker and more robust hair.

2. **Prevention of Scalp Issues:** Common scalp conditions such as dandruff, seborrheic dermatitis, and dryness can impede hair growth and negatively affect the hair's overall health. Regular and effective scalp care can help minimize these problems. For example, addressing excessive dryness or oiliness through proper scalp hygiene and moisturizing can stabilize conditions like flaking and irritation.

3. **Enhanced Hair Appearance:** A clean, nourished scalp directly contributes to healthier, shinier hair. The condition of the scalp significantly impacts the quality of the hair that grows from it. By maintaining a healthy scalp, you can achieve hair that is not only visually appealing but also soft, manageable, and less prone to breakage.

Proper Cleansing Techniques

Cleansing the scalp is a vital aspect of hair care, especially for natural textures prone to dryness and product build-up. The goal is to remove dirt, excess oils, and residues while preserving the natural oils that keep the scalp and hair healthy. Here are some effective cleansing techniques:

1. **Frequency of Washing:** The frequency of scalp washing depends on individual hair types and lifestyles. For natural textured hair, washing once a week or every 10-14 days is generally recommended, depending on the styling method. Over-washing can strip the hair of its natural oils, while infrequent washing can lead to build-up and scalp issues. Adjust the washing schedule based on your scalp's condition and personal preference.

2. **Choosing the Right Shampoo:** Select a sulfate-free shampoo to avoid harsh chemicals that strip natural oils from the scalp. Sulfates, known for their strong cleansing properties, can be too harsh for natural hair, causing dryness and irritation. Instead, opt for shampoos with gentle ingredients that cleanse without disrupting the scalp's natural balance.

   Avoid coconut and honey-infused products, as their small molecular structure can penetrate the hair shaft, blocking out moisture. Limit the use of cleansing shampoos and detox treatments to a maximum of three times per year, as these products can worsen moisture deficiency in hair that is already malnourished.

3. Massage Techniques: Incorporate gentle scalp massages during washing to stimulate blood flow and promote relaxation. Use the pads of your fingers—not your nails—to avoid scratching the scalp. Massage in circular motions to enhance circulation and help the shampoo work more effectively. A 5- to 10-second massage provides enough friction to release build-up from the scalp, loosening dirt, product residues, and dead skin cells.

4. Rinsing Thoroughly: Thoroughly rinse out all shampoo and conditioner to avoid residue build-up, which can irritate the scalp and weigh down the hair. Saturate the hair with water before applying shampoo to help relax and elongate curls. Use lukewarm water for rinsing, as hot water can exacerbate dryness and irritation, while cold water helps to seal the hair cuticle.

5. Conditioning and Moisturizing: After cleansing, apply a conditioner to replenish moisture and maintain softness. Distribute the conditioner evenly by brushing through your hair. For enhanced hydration, always follow up with a leave-in conditioner, even if a scalp treatment has been used. This final step ensures ongoing moisture retention and helps maintain overall hair health.

Product Recommendations

Choosing the right products is essential for maintaining a healthy scalp and natural hair. Here are some recommended product types to consider:

1. **Clarifying Shampoos:** Clarifying shampoos are ideal for removing product buildup and residue but should be used sparingly—no more than three times a year. These shampoos provide a deep cleanse but can be

drying if overused. Choose formulas with gentle ingredients and free of harsh chemicals. Avoid clarifying shampoos entirely if your hair is experiencing dryness, as they can exacerbate breakage.

2. **Moisturizing Shampoos:** Moisturizing shampoos formulated with hydrating ingredients such as aloe vera, glycerin, or emollients are a must-have for Afro hair. These products help maintain a healthy moisture balance in the scalp and hair, reducing dryness while enhancing softness and manageability.

3. **Scalp Treatments:** Incorporating scalp treatments into your routine can greatly benefit scalp health. Consider exfoliating scrubs to remove dead skin cells and promote a clean, healthy scalp environment. Soothing oils, such as tea tree or peppermint oil, offer antimicrobial properties and can invigorate the scalp while boosting blood circulation. These treatments support overall scalp vitality and help foster optimal hair growth.

4. **Conditioners and Deep Conditioners:** Hydration-focused conditioners are key to addressing most natural hair needs. For added nourishment, deep conditioning treatments provide intensive hydration and repair, improving hair health and elasticity. Avoid protein or keratin-infused conditioners if your hair is dry, as these can increase brittleness and lead to further breakage.

5. **Leave-In Conditioners and Oils:** Leave-in conditioners and natural oils like jojoba or argan oil help maintain moisture, reduce frizz, and enhance shine. Use these products sparingly to avoid a greasy feel. Typically, a nickel-sized amount is sufficient—rub it between your hands before patting it gently through your hair, then use a brush to distribute evenly.

Scalp health and hygiene are pivotal to achieving and maintaining beautiful natural hair. A healthy scalp supports optimal hair growth, prevents common scalp issues, and enhances the overall appearance of your hair.

By adopting proper cleansing techniques, choosing the right products, and incorporating effective scalp care practices, you can nurture both scalp and hair health. As a stylist, mastering these practices allows you to provide superior care and guidance to clients, empowering them to achieve their hair care goals and embrace their natural beauty with confidence.

LESSON 2:
CLEANSING AND CONDITIONING

Cleansing and conditioning are essential steps in a natural hair care routine. Proper cleansing removes impurities and product buildup, while conditioning restores moisture, softness, and manageability. This lesson provides expert insights on the best practices for washing and conditioning natural hair and offers guidance on selecting the right products based on hair type and needs.

Best Practices for Washing Natural Hair

1. **Determine the Appropriate Frequency:** The frequency of washing natural hair depends on individual hair type, scalp condition, and styling preferences. Typically, washing every 7–14 days is recommended for natural hair not in a protective style. For hair in a protective style, shampooing may not be necessary for up to 8 weeks if the scalp is properly prepped beforehand.

   Washing too frequently can strip the hair of its natural oils, leading to dryness, while infrequent washing may cause product buildup and scalp issues. Tailor your washing routine to your scalp's needs and your hair's response to cleansing. For protective styles, focus on maintaining a hydrated scalp rather than regular shampooing.

2. **Co-wash Treatments:** Before shampooing, some recommend using a pre-shampoo treatment or applying oil to the hair to help protect against the drying effects of shampoo and add moisture. However, while co-washing (using conditioner to cleanse hair) can help with detangling, it does not effectively break down oils and dirt on the scalp.

Over-reliance on co-washing can lead to clogged hair follicles, buildup, and scalp irritation, potentially causing issues like inflammation or scalp acne. Use co-wash treatments sparingly and ensure proper scalp cleansing with shampoo when needed.

3. **Choose a Sulfate-Free Shampoo:** Sulfates, such as sodium lauryl sulfate, are harsh detergents found in many shampoos that can strip natural hair of essential oils and cause dryness. Opt for sulfate-free shampoos formulated with mild surfactants and natural ingredients to maintain moisture balance while effectively cleansing.

   If your hair often feels dry and resistant to moisture, avoid products rich in coconut, honey, protein, or keratin. While these ingredients fill gaps in the hair strand to "strengthen" it, they can block moisture absorption, leading to dryness and breakage.

4. **Apply Shampoo to the Scalp:** When washing, focus on applying shampoo directly to the scalp. Shampoo naturally spreads from the scalp to the ends, but it does not travel effectively in the reverse direction. The primary purpose of shampooing is to cleanse the scalp.

   Gently massage the shampoo into your scalp with your fingertips to lift dirt, excess oil, and buildup. Avoid using your nails, as this can cause irritation or damage. Rinse thoroughly to remove all impurities, preparing your hair for conditioning.

5. **Rinse Thoroughly:** Thoroughly rinsing out shampoo is critical to preventing scalp irritation and product buildup. Use lukewarm water to rinse, as this helps open the hair cuticles for more effective cleansing. Follow with a cool rinse to close the cuticles and seal in moisture.

6. **Avoid Over-Processing:** To protect your hair from over-drying and damage, avoid using very hot water or

excessive amounts of shampoo. Similarly, avoid vigorous scrubbing, which can cause breakage. Instead, focus on gentle, effective cleansing techniques to ensure your hair and scalp are clean and healthy without unnecessary stress.

Best Practices for Conditioning Natural Hair

1. **Select the Right Conditioner:** Conditioning is crucial for replenishing moisture and maintaining hair health. Choose a conditioner specifically formulated to provide your hair with optimal hydration. For natural hair, opt for a moisturizing conditioner containing ingredients like jojoba oil, avocado oil, or glycerin, as these provide the nourishment needed to keep hair soft and manageable. Avoid products that focus on strengthening, such as those containing honey, coconut, protein, or keratin, as they may not address dryness effectively.

2. **Apply Conditioner to Hair:** After rinsing out shampoo, apply conditioner evenly from root to tip. Use a detangling or paddle brush to distribute the product evenly and gently detangle your hair.

3. **Deep Conditioning Treatments:** Make deep conditioning treatments a part of your routine at least once a month. These treatments deliver intense hydration and repair, which are particularly beneficial for natural hair prone to dryness and damage. Look for deep conditioners that focus on intense moisture penetration. Avoid strengthening ingredients like keratin, honey, or silk proteins, as they can exacerbate dryness rather than resolve it.

4. **Use Heat for Better Penetration:** To boost the effectiveness of your deep conditioning treatment, apply heat. Options include using a hooded dryer, a heated cap, or wrapping your hair in a warm towel. Heat

helps open the hair cuticles, allowing the conditioner to penetrate deeply for better results. If using a dryer, limit the session to 20 minutes. Without a dryer, leave the conditioner on for up to 45 minutes under a plastic cap. In either case, use a steam bonnet under the cap.

5. **Rinse with Cool Water:** After conditioning, rinse your hair thoroughly with cool water. This helps close the cuticles, locking in moisture and enhancing shine and smoothness. Ensure all conditioner is rinsed out to prevent residue buildup, which can weigh down the hair and lead to dullness. A thorough rinse will also ensure the scalp remains free of product buildup.

Product Selection Based on Hair Type and Needs

1. **Identify Your Hair Type:** Understanding your hair type is essential for selecting the right products. Natural hair can range from wavy to tightly coiled, with each type having its own unique needs. Determine whether your hair is fine, medium, or coarse, and assess its porosity (low or high). Hair porosity affects how well your hair absorbs and retains moisture, which influences your product choices. This knowledge will also help you apply products more effectively. If a product doesn't seem to work for your hair, it may be that you're not using it correctly. For some textures, you may need to dampen your hair after product application to achieve the desired styling results.

2. **Hydrating Products:** For dry or brittle hair, look for hydrating products that provide deep moisture. Ingredients such as aloe vera, glycerin, and butylene glycol are excellent for hydration and improving elasticity. Moisturizing shampoos and conditioners help maintain softness and prevent breakage. Moisture is often the #1 missing piece in the equation for healthy, vibrant hair.

3. **Protein Treatments:** If your hair is damaged or lacks strength, avoid rushing into protein treatments. While products containing hydrolyzed proteins like keratin or silk proteins can offer benefits, they can also further damage your hair if overused. Protein is essentially a filler that prevents moisture from penetrating the hair shaft, which may contribute to hair damage if not used properly. Overuse of protein treatments can cause hair to become stiff and prone to breakage. If you've experienced weak or damaged hair, protein buildup might be a factor. It typically takes about 3 to 4 months for this buildup to be removed naturally and allow moisture to enter the hair shaft again.

4. **Detangling Products:** or hair prone to tangling, choose conditioners or leave-in products with good slip to make the detangling process easier. Ingredients like marshmallow root or slippery elm are helpful in reducing breakage and making the process smoother.

5. **Scalp Care Products:** If you experience scalp issues like dryness or dandruff, look for products designed specifically for scalp care. Ingredients such as tea tree oil, salicylic acid, or peppermint oil can help address these concerns and promote a healthier scalp environment. However, keep in mind that these ingredients may exfoliate the top layers of skin, so flaking may occur initially.

Cleansing and conditioning are the foundational steps in maintaining the health and beauty of natural, textured hair. By following best practices for washing and conditioning, and selecting the right products based on your hair's specific needs, you can ensure your hair stays clean, moisturized, and manageable. Whether you're a stylist providing expert care to clients or an individual caring for your own natural hair, understanding these principles will help you achieve optimal results and enhance the overall health and appearance of your hair.

LESSON 3:
MOISTURE RETENTION TECHNIQUES

Hydration Methods for Natural Hair

1. **Understanding Hair Porosity:** Hair porosity refers to the hair's ability to absorb and retain moisture. There are three main types: low, medium, and high porosity. Low porosity hair has tightly closed cuticles, making it difficult for moisture to penetrate, while high porosity hair has gaps in the cuticles, allowing moisture to escape easily. Medium porosity hair has a balanced ability to absorb and retain moisture. Identifying your hair's porosity helps in selecting the right hydration methods and products.

2. **Hydrating with Water:** Water is the most essential and natural hydrator for hair. Incorporate water-based products into your routine, such as leave-in conditioners and sprays, to provide ongoing moisture. Regularly misting your hair with water or using a hydrating spray throughout the day can help maintain moisture levels.

3. **Using Moisturizing Products:** Choose hair care products specifically designed to add and retain moisture. Look for moisturizers that contain ingredients like glycerin, aloe vera, and avocado, and avoid sulfates. These ingredients help attract and lock moisture into the hair, enhancing hydration. Moisturizing conditioners, creams, and oils are great for replenishing and maintaining moisture levels.

4. **Incorporating Leave-In Conditioners:** Leave-in conditioners are an excellent way to provide continuous moisture and manageability. Apply a leave-in conditioner after washing your hair to help detangle and hydrate. Choose formulas enriched with humectants

like butylene glycol, which draw moisture from the air and into the hair.

5. **Deep Conditioning Treatments:** Deep conditioning is a crucial part of a moisture retention regimen. Use deep conditioners or hair masks once a month to provide intensive hydration and repair. Opt for products that offer a balance of moisture and protein to strengthen and hydrate the hair. Ingredients like cetearyl alcohol, avocado oil, and olive oil are ideal for deep conditioning treatments.

Moisture-Protein Balance Scale With Healthy Hydration Phase

Scale value	Hair Condition	Hair Behavior	Product Recommendations
0-2	Severe Protein Buildup	Hair is extremely stiff and brittle, lacking flexibility. Snaps immediately when stretched.	Use deep moisture treatments, hydrating masks, and avoid protein-heavy products.
3-5	Moderate Protein	Moderate Protein Buildup. Hair has some flexibility but still feels stiff and dry.	Increase hydration with deep conditioners and moisture-based leave-ins.
6-8	Healthy Hydration Phase	Hair is well-hydrated and close to ideal, but may need minor structural adjustments for resilience.	Maintain hydration with occasional strengthening treatments for balance.
9-11	Balanced Hair Health	Hair has a perfect balance of moisture and protein. It stretches before breaking and feels strong yet flexible.	Continue using a mix of moisture and protein to maintain elasticity and strength.
12-14	Weak/Dry Hair (Product Barrier)	Hair feels overly soft and lacks internal support, making it prone to breakage. Needs moisture.	Use a cleansing shampoo to remove buildup and follow with moisture-rich products, avoiding protein treatments. Remove oil.

Too Much Protein   **Balanced**   Needs Moisture
Moisture-Protein Balance Scale With Healthy Hydration Phase

1-2 (Severe Protein Buildup)   3-5 (Moderate Protein Buildup)   6-8 (Healthy Hydration Phase)   9-11 (Balanced Hair Health)   12-14 (Weak/Dry Hair - Product Barrier)

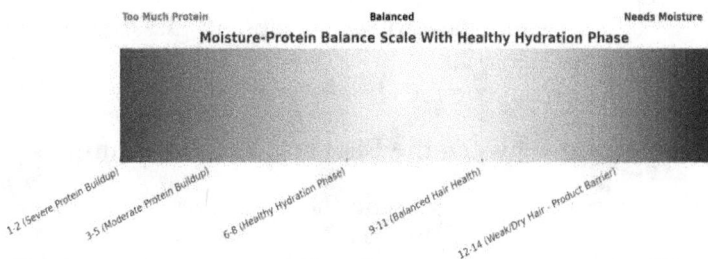

1-2 (Severe Protein Buildup) → Hair is stiff, brittle, and lacks flexibility. Needs deep moisture treatments.

3-5 (Moderate Protein Buildup) → Hair is slightly stiff and prone to breakage. Increase hydration.

6-8 (Healthy Hydration Phase) → Hair is close to ideal, needing only minor structural adjustments.

9-11 (Balanced Hair Health) → Hair has a perfect moisture-protein ratio with proper elasticity and strength.

12-14 (Weak/Dry Hair - Product Barrier) → Hair feels overly soft but lacks internal support, needing cleansing and moisture.

How to Perform the Shampoo-Based Moisture-Protein Test

This test helps determine whether your hair has too much protein, too much moisture, or a balanced moisture-protein ratio using just your shampoo and fingertips.

Step-by-Step Guide

1. **Prep Your Hair**

   - Wet your hair thoroughly with warm water to ensure it's fully saturated.
   - Use your regular moisturizing shampoo (not a clarifying shampoo).

2. **First Shampoo Application**

- Apply shampoo to your scalp and massage as you normally would.
- Rinse out completely with warm water.

3. Testing Between the First and Second Shampoo

Now, perform the finger slide and squeak test:

- ○ Slide your thumb and index finger down a few strands of wet hair to check for resistance.
- ○ Rub your thumb and index finger together and observe the sensation.

Shampoo-Based Moisture-Protein Test

	What It Means	Hair Condition	What to Do
Fingers feel rough while feeling ridges on fingers	Hair cuticles are too stiff, indicating a lack of flexibility and excess protein buildup.	Severe Protein Buildup (0-2 on Scale)	Use deep hydration treatments and avoid protein-heavy products.
Fingers squeak loudly when rubbed together	Hair resists moisture, feeling slightly stiff but not excessively brittle.	Moderate Protein Buildup (3-5 on Scale)	Increase moisture-rich products to soften and improve elasticity.
Fingers start to squeak slightly	Hair has a healthy balance of moisture and protein, allowing it to stretch before breaking.	Healthy Hydration Phase (6-8 on Scale)	Maintain hydration with occasional strengthening treatments.
Fingers slide smoothly, no squeak	Hair is well-hydrated but may have minor structural gaps affecting strength.	Balanced Hair Health (9-11 on Scale)	Continue a mix of moisture and protein to reinforce elasticity.
Fingers feel soft but greasy	Product is too heavy, creating a barrier that blocks moisture instead of allowing absorption.	Weak/Dry Hair (12-14 on Scale)	Use a cleansing shampoo to remove buildup and follow with moisture-rich products, avoiding protein treatments

Product Recommendations

1. **Water-Based Moisturizers**: Water-based moisturizers are essential for hydration. Products like *Design Essentials Almond Avocado Daily Moisturizing Lotion* and *Moisture Love Moisture and Style Cream* are excellent choices. These products contain ingredients that help lock in moisture and provide long-lasting hydration. Avoid brands like Cantu and Shea Moisture, as I've noticed that many cases of product-related damage come from these two lines.

2. **Hydrating Sprays**: Hydrating sprays, such as *Jamaican Mango Lime No More Itch Gro Spray* and *Design Essentials Curl Revitalizing Spray*, are perfect for refreshing and adding moisture to dry hair. These sprays can be used between wash days to maintain hydration and manageability.

3. **Deep Conditioners:** For deep conditioning, consider products like the *Doo Gro Reconstructive Mask* (green or blue) and *Differ Jojoba Deep Conditioning Mask*. These masks are formulated to deeply penetrate the hair shaft, delivering essential moisture and nutrients.

4. **Oils for Moisture Sealing:** Natural oils, such as argan oil, castor oil, and jojoba oil, are fantastic for sealing in moisture. Oils help lock in the hydration provided by other products and form a protective barrier against moisture loss. Use oils sparingly to avoid buildup and prevent weighing down the hair. In my opinion, coconut oil is a "no-no" for natural hair.

5. **Leave-In Conditioners:** Effective leave-in conditioners, such as *Paul Mitchell The Conditioner* and *Moisture Love Leave-In Conditioning Serum*, provide continuous moisture and help manage hair throughout the week. They also assist in detangling and reducing breakage.

Sealing in Moisture for Lasting Hydration

1. **The LOC and LCO Methods:** The LOC (Liquid, Oil, Cream) and LCO (Liquid, Cream, Oil) methods are popular techniques for sealing in moisture. The LOC method involves applying a liquid (such as water or leave-in conditioner), followed by an oil (like castor or olive oil), and then a cream (such as a styling cream or butter). The LCO method, on the other hand, starts with the liquid, followed by a cream, and then an oil. Both methods effectively lock in moisture and keep hair hydrated. Both methods work well, but I recommend using the LOC method if styling is done on dry hair with a mousse or gel, and the LCO method if styling is done on wet hair with mousse or gel.

2. **Oil Sealing:** Applying oils to your hair after moisturizing is an effective way to seal in hydration. Oils create a barrier that prevents moisture from escaping, ensuring your hair stays hydrated for longer periods. For the best results, apply a small amount of oil to damp hair and distribute it evenly.

3. **Layering Products:** Layering products is another great technique for enhancing moisture retention. Start with a water-based leave-in conditioner, followed by a moisturizing cream or butter, and finish by sealing with oil. This method effectively traps moisture and provides lasting hydration.

4. **Protective Styles:** Incorporating protective styles into your routine can help retain moisture by reducing exposure to environmental factors that cause dryness. Styles such as braids, twists, or buns help preserve moisture levels and minimize breakage—as long as you prep before you protect.

5. **Hydration Maintenance:** Maintaining hydration requires consistency. Ensure your hair is regularly

moisturized, and avoid skipping hydration treatments. Track your hair's moisture needs and adjust your routine accordingly.

6. **Avoid Over-Manipulation:** Excessive manipulation or handling of hair can lead to moisture loss and breakage. Minimize the temperature of heat styling tools and avoid tight hairstyles that can stress both the hair and scalp. Focus on gentle handling and protective measures to prevent breakage.

Mastering moisture retention is essential for achieving and maintaining vibrant, healthy natural hair. By understanding the importance of hydration and employing effective techniques and products, you can ensure that your hair remains well-moisturized, soft, and resilient. Whether you're caring for your own natural hair or providing services for clients, these strategies will help you achieve optimal moisture levels and enhance the overall health and appearance of natural textured hair.

QUIZ

Lesson 1: Scalp Health and Hygiene

1. Question

Why is scalp health important for maintaining healthy hair?

a) It reduces dandruff.

b) It promotes better hair growth.

c) It improves hair color retention.

d) It shortens hair styling time.

Answer: b) It promotes better hair growth.

2. Question

Which of the following is a proper technique for cleansing the scalp?

a) Scrubbing with your nails to remove buildup.

b) Using a brush to exfoliate the scalp.

c) Gently massaging the scalp with fingertips.

d) Applying shampoo to the scalp directly.

Answer: c) Gently massaging the scalp with fingertips. And d) is correct as well.

3. Question

Which type of product is recommended for people with a sensitive scalp?

a) Sulfate-free shampoo.

b) Gel-based conditioners.

c) Heavy oil-based cleansers.

d) Dry shampoo.

Answer: a) Sulfate-free shampoo.

Lesson 2: Cleansing and Conditioning

1. Question

What should you consider when selecting a conditioner for natural hair?

a) Hair type, porosity, and moisture needs.

b) The scent and color of the product.

c) The price of the conditioner.

d) The thickness of the product.

Answer: a) Hair type, porosity, and moisture needs.

2. Question

Which of the following is NOT a recommended conditioning practice for natural hair?

a) Deep conditioning once a week.

b) Leaving regular conditioner in for more than an hour.

c) Applying conditioner from mid-shaft to ends.

d) Using leave-in conditioner for extra moisture.

Answer: c) Applying conditioner from mid-shaft to ends.

Lesson 3: Moisture Retention Techniques

1. Question

Which of the following is a key hydration method for natural hair?

a) Using a clarifying shampoo weekly.

b) Regularly applying water-based moisturizers.

c) Applying heavy oils daily.

d) Using a heated styling tool after washing.

Answer: b) Regularly applying water-based moisturizers.

2. Question

Which type of product helps seal in moisture after applying a water-based moisturizer?

a) Cream-based conditioner.

b) Clarifying shampoo.

c) Light oils like jojoba or almond oil.

d) Alcohol-based styling gel.

Answer: c) Light oils like jojoba or almond oil.

3. Question

What is the "LOC" method in natural hair care?

a) Layering Oil first, then Conditioner.

b) Using Leave-in, Oil, and Cream to retain moisture.

c) Locking moisture with a heavy butter or wax product.

d) Leaving conditioner in overnight for maximum hydration.

Answer: b) Using Leave-in, Oil, and Cream to retain moisture

4. Question

Which of the following is a good product recommendation for lasting hydration in natural hair?

a) Sulfate shampoo.

b) Using a leave-in conditioner.

c) High alcohol content mousse.

d) Dry shampoo with added fragrance.

Answer: Using a leave-in conditioner.

CLOSING NOTE

Your hair isn't "hard to manage."

It just needs the right kind of nourishment.

Master moisture—and you master one of the most
powerful parts of your journey.